Watersports Safety and Emergency First Aid

D1555688

*A***FALCON**GUIDE®

Watersports Safety and Emergency First Aid

A Handbook for Boaters, Anglers, Kayakers, River Runners, and Surfriders

Christopher Van Tilburg, M.D.

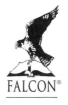

FALCON®

GUILFORD, CONNECTICUT
AN IMPRINT OF THE GLOBE PEQUOT PRESS

A FALCON GUIDE ®

Copyright © 2002 by Christopher Van Tilburg

Text design by Lisa Reneson
Illustrations by Diane Blasius

Library of Congress Cataloging-in-Publication Data
Van Tilburg, Christopher.
  Watersports safety and emergency first aid: a handbook for boaters, anglers, sea kayakers, and river runners / by Christopher Van Tilburg.—1st ed.
    p. cm.—(A Falcon Guide)
Includes bibliographical references and index.
ISBN 0-7627-2353-X (pbk.)
1. Aquatic sports—Safety measures. 2. Boats and boating—Safety measures. 3. First aid in illness and injury. I. Title: Water sports safety and emergency first aid. II. Title. III. Series.
GV770.6.V36. 2002
363.14—dc21   2002019587

Manufactured in the United States of America
First Edition/First Printing

Table of Contents

Introduction

You're surfing a remote point break, kayaking your local stream, or casting your fly rod in the ocean. Whatever the case, watersports are thrilling and wondrous, peaceful and adventuresome. But they can also be dangerous. We all hope that we won't need to use survival skills on the water, and that our emergency equipment will remain forever stashed in our drybags or tackle boxes. In dangerous circumstances, however, refined survival skills and a well-stocked emergency pack can save your life.

Water emergencies and survival situations vary enormously. There are different weather and water conditions in different places. Activities differ, as well; whether it's surfing, diving, snorkeling, fishing, or kayaking, different sports require different gear and have distinct safety issues. The differences in gear start with the watercraft used for different sports. Snorkelers and anglers may not even use boats;

personal boats are used in sports like kayaking; surfers, kiteboarders, and windsurfers use boards; and boats vary in size from little canoes to big sailboats equipped with high-tech navigational equipment. I've written this book to cover a broad range of sports, conditions, waterways, and watercraft.

A comprehensive guide to watersports safety would require volumes. This book is a brief introduction to a very large subject, a careful selection of basic background information and useful tips. If you'd like more information than I can present here, refer to appendix A for a list of resources.

A Note on Zero-Impact Watersports

You're probably familiar with the Leave No Trace ethic of minimizing environmental impacts. By paddling softly and swimming gently, we allow plants and animals to flourish, keep the land and waterways pristine for future visitors, and help prevent degradation of the environment. *Leave No Trace: Minimum Impact Outdoor Recreation* by Will Harmon (Falcon, 1997) is the official manual of the American Hiking Society. Although it mainly covers travel on land, it contains excellent information for watersports and coastal and riverine environments.

Keep these basic zero-impact principles in mind when you travel on water:

■ Don't toss waste or food scraps overboard. Take out everything you take in, even toilet paper. Some riverine recreation activities, such as Grand Canyon river trips, require a portable toilet so that all human waste is carried out.

■ Keep your gear stowed or lashed so that it doesn't get washed overboard.

■ Whenever practical, build your land camp at least 300 feet from a stream, ocean, or lake. Cooking, bathing, using a latrine, and sleeping should all take place at least that distance from the water. Make sure you're well above the high-water mark or high tide. Don't throw cooking water, urine, or bathing water back into waterways. Use a small hole for wastewater or scatter it over a broad area on land.

■ Use caution when entering and exiting water. Banks and beaches can be especially fragile. Plants and animals use this transition zone as a vital link between land and water environments. Avoid fragile animal and plant habitats, such as beaver dams, tidepools, coral reefs, or streamside meadows.

■ Make sure you aren't following a route too difficult for your ability. When in trouble, a novice on an expert route tends to make the way easier by damaging water ecosystems. For example, a canoeist encountering rapids too difficult for his or her skills might be forced to drag the boat along the shore or through the shallows, but that can disrupt fish or plant habitat significantly by stirring up dirt or destroying stream banks.

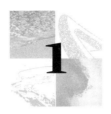

Water Safety Basics

Where to Begin

Watersports safety is a huge topic, encompassing everything from safety to first aid, prevention to survival. It can seem pretty overwhelming. But there's a good place to start: Become familiar with the general hazards of the water world. This is the first step toward minimizing your risk of a serious mishap. Test yourself: You should know and understand the dangers listed below in the area where you're headed. Weather hazards can include fog, rain, sleet, hail, lightning, thunderstorms, wind, sun, and others. Water conditions vary depending on the environment: open ocean, surf beaches, or inland waterways.

- Open ocean poses particular dangers with wind waves, swells, and currents, all commonly made more serious if you're in a remote location offshore.

- Surf beaches have waves, rip currents, back-

wash, shore break, littoral currents, sandbars,
tidepools, and flotsam.

■ Inland streams and lakes can have rapids, submerged rocks, deadheads, fast currents, fish
and animals, eddies, waterfalls, and human-
made structures such as dams and bridges.

When learning water safety, there are some
general ideas you can follow to minimize your
risk for accidents. First, start at home. Swim
regularly to stay in shape for watersports emergencies. Keep your muscles and cardiovascular
system in excellent shape. Know your gear, too:
Make sure it's in excellent working condition
and learn how to use everything in your emergency pack, especially survival and first-aid
items.

Second, learn water safety and survival from
a certified instructor and detailed books on the
subject. Regular practice should include dry-
land training.

Third, use caution and good judgment when
out and about. Don't let your energy, food, or
fluid reserves get low. Keep your spirits high,
too. Don't let your body or mind get tired or
groggy. You're much more vulnerable to disaster when you're tired, cold, and wet, are in a sit-

uation too difficult for your skill level, or are in a position for which you don't have the proper equipment.

Fourth, leave a float plan with someone you trust. An example is listed in appendix B. Always check the marine and weather forecasts and have a contingency plan for foul weather or rough water. Don't be afraid to turn around at the dock and go home if water or weather conditions are unsafe.

Getting the Scoop on Weather and Water Conditions

Weather and water conditions are the two biggest variables when planning a trip. From sparkling sunshine to a torrential downpour, things can change instantly. There are lots of ways you can get current conditions and the forecast. You probably already check with your local television, radio, or Internet Web site. The best place for up-to-date info is from the two branches of the National Oceanic and Atmospheric Association (NOAA): the National Weather Service (NWS) and the National Ocean Service (NOS). These agencies give current weather and water conditions as well as short- and long-range forecasts in a number of formats: Radio and Internet are the most common and easiest to access. There may be a local phone number in your area for recorded up-to-date information.

On the Internet, the National Weather Service is at www.nws.noaa.gov and the National Ocean Service is at www.nos.noaa.gov. The U.S. Coast Guard site posts water, weather, and general boating safety information and can be found at www.uscgboating.org. Mark these pages on your "favorites" list. You don't necessarily need to spend a lot of time surfing these sites, but check them to learn the weather and water patterns and conditions in your area.

A number of radio services give up-to-the-minute information. If you carry a weather, FM, or VHF radio with you, you can get current data anytime.

■ In the United States, NOAA weather radio is on one of three frequencies, depending on your location: 162.55 megahertz (MHz), 162.40 MHz, or 162.475 MHz.

■ In Canada, weather is broadcast at 161.65 MHz.

■ On FM radio, the NWS broadcasts hourly weather at 5, 10, and 15 MHz.

■ The U.S. Coast Guard broadcasts weather information on VHF marine radio on channel 22A; storm warnings are usually initially posted on channel 16. On single side bands (SSB), they are on channel 2670 kilohertz (kHz) after an initial storm warning on 2182 kHz.

NOAA categorizes storm warnings as follows:

■ **Small craft advisory** forecasts winds from 18 to 33 knots with seas that can be hazardous to small boats.

■ **Gale warning** forecasts winds from 34 to 47 knots.

■ **Storm warning** forecasts winds of 48 knots or greater.

■ **Hurricane warning** forecasts winds over 64 knots.

■ **Special marine warnings** can be put out with thunderstorms or squalls, usually with winds greater than 35 knots.

Personal Flotation Device

Personal flotation devices (PFDs) are vital for boating safety. They're required equipment for boats in most states. They come in a multitude of sizes and shapes for different people and applications. When choosing a PFD, make sure it fits—it should be snug but comfortable. And make sure it's readily available, not stashed at the bottom of the hold under piles of scuba gear. PFDs should be approved by the Coast Guard in the United States or other certifying agencies abroad. There are several types of personal flotation devices as classified by the U.S. Coast Guard.

■ **Type I** is called an **offshore life jacket.** These are designed to float unconscious swimmers faceup in rough water. They can be difficult to find for young kids and are bulky.

■ **Type II** is called a **near-shore buoyant vest.** These are general-use life jackets that will float many unconscious swimmers faceup in water. For kids and infants, Type II PFDs should come with a groin strap and an extra flotation pad behind the child's head and neck. These are the most common PFDs and probably the best for multipurpose use.

■ **Type III,** a **flotation aid,** is designed to be comfortable for long periods of activity such as when waterskiing, fishing, sailing, rafting, or kayaking. These are best for people with superior swimming skills traveling in relatively calm waters.

■ **Type IV** is a **throwable device** such as a life ring or a floatable seat cushion. These are usually on boats for emergency rescue when someone who can swim needs to be rescued. They're not designed for use as a primary PFD.

■ **Type V** is classified as a **special-use device** such as certain wetsuits, survival suits, or sport-specific vests such as those for windsurfing, whitewater kayaking, or waterskiing. These don't have nearly as much flotation as a Type I, II, or III, and typically aren't recommended for the general public.

Personal Protective Clothing

Clothing is another important, often misunderstood and undervalued piece of survival equipment. Yes, clothing is equipment. It's widely variable, depending on your activity and the weather and water conditions. Always make sure you have extra clothes and prepare for all conditions. You don't have to spend tons of money, but get good-quality gear. It will perform better and last longer. But beware:

Expensive models of clothing sometimes have bells and whistles you don't need.

Foul-Weather Clothing

Rain gear is a must for most watersports; it should be windproof and waterproof. Make sure you have a jacket with a hood and pants you can fit over your regular pants. A large-brimmed rain hat will keep your head dry and, more importantly, keep water from running down your back. Knee-high rubber boots should be able to tuck under your pants so the boots don't fill with water. If you're paddling, it helps to have tight cuffs at the ankles and wrists to help seal out water. Some rainwear specifically designed for kayaking, rafting, or canoeing has just such gaskets on the neck, ankles, and wrists.

For insulation, polypropylene and polyester are the standard. Synthetic clothing is light, durable, dries quickly, and retains some insulation properties when wet. Down, wool, and similar materials generally aren't suitable for watersports. When wet, they're heavy and lose much of their insulating properties (especially down), and they take a long time to dry.

Wetsuits, Drysuits, and Survival Suits

A wetsuit is mandatory for any cold-water activity in which you'll be in the water for any length of time, such as surfing or diving. They have different designs, materials, and construction, depending on the sport or use. They come in a variety of thicknesses, ranging from 1 to 6 millimeters. The warmest suit is a long-sleeved, long-armed 6-millimeter-thick dive or surf suit. The more common suit is 3 to 4 millimeters thick with long legs and either long or short sleeves. Some minimalist suits are a T-shirt and shorts. When in cold water, you should consider wearing a neoprene hood, booties, and gloves, too.

Drysuits are warmer than wetsuits and are usually reserved for special situations and very cold water. You can wear bulky warm clothes underneath that will stay dry.

Survival suits are foam suits designed for offshore, open-ocean travel to be used in emergency situations by oceangoing vessels on long trips.

Sun Clothes

Sun protection is also extremely important, whether you're in the pool, at the beach, or on the river. We know a bad burn in childhood increases risks for skin cancer later in life. And it's so easily preventable! Skimpy swimsuits don't offer much protection from ultraviolet rays. Sun-protective clothing, on the other hand, doesn't wear off like sunscreen, and you can use it again and again.

Tightly knit polyester and cotton, found in standard T-shirts, probably have a sun protection factor (SPF) of around 10. Surf, dive, and snorkel shops usually sell rash guards—thin spandex T-shirts that provide protection from the sun. Some companies make sun clothing designed for fishing or adventure travel that has an SPF higher than 10. These are made of tightly woven nylon that blocks the sun, and dry quickly when wet.

Remember to get long-sleeved shirts and long pants for maximum protection. Wear a wide-brimmed sun hat or a cap that has an attached scarf to protect the back of your neck and ears. Make sure the hat has a strap and is washable—you'll sweat in it. Eye protection is important, too: Use good-quality sunglasses that block out ultraviolet light. Wear watersports goggles when in the water kayaking, surfing, or windsurfing. Polarized lenses help

WATER SAFETY BASICS ■ 11

diminish glare, especially at sea, but they also lessen definition of waves and swells somewhat.

Helmets

Always wear a brain bucket when rafting, kayaking, surfing, windsurfing, or involved in other adventure sports. It's best to get a helmet designed for the respective sport; specialty helmets are now available for windsurfing, surfing, kayaking, and other watersports. Your lid should be snug but not uncomfortable. It should have a waterproof chin strap, lots of padding, and good visibility.

Footwear

Footwear is probably the least considered piece of equipment, but just as valuable as anything you own. If your feet are cold or injured, you're at a significant disadvantage in a survival situation; you may even be unable to get to safety. Your shoes or

Hint: Use an old pair of shoes—they will get trashed. For extra warmth, wear neoprene socks with the shoes. Tall rubber boots or waders work great for fishing or exploring tidepools. You can also buy waterproof overboots that fit over light tennis shoes, but these can be cumbersome to put on and walk in. For surfing, sailboarding, diving, or snorkeling, choose neoprene booties.

boots should be durable and warm—especially when wading, snorkeling, or tidepooling—so that you don't injure your feet on rocks, coral, or barnacles. Amphibious shoes such as those designed for kayaking or canyoneering work well to keep feet warm or protect them when walking in water. Canvas tennis shoes or light-weight hiking shoes work well for wading and are an inexpensive alternative. Rubber soles provide traction on slippery wet rocks.

Electronics

Electronics are ubiquitous in our world now; most people don't go into the wilds without at least a headlamp. We have gadgets with so many high-tech bells and whistles to help with our sports and survival that the instruction manuals are like small books. Electronics can be tremendously helpful, but they're also unreli-able in some situations. Drop them overboard: useless. Dead batteries: useless. Also, some units that require land- or satellite-based links can be inoperable if the receiving stations fail if you're traveling in dense fog or among tall hills. Store all your electronics in padded watertight plastic cases such as those made by Pelican or Otter Box—available at many outdoor and marine supply stores.

Global positioning system (GPS) units, compasses, altimeters, cell phones, and, most recently, satellite phones are popular handheld devices that aid in navigation and signaling. These are discussed later on, under "Signaling" and "Emergency Navigation." Other devices that you'll find only on larger boats include:

■ Emergency Position Indicating Radio Beacon (EPIRB). Several models of these beacons are available, linked to satellite and land stations.

■ Global Maritime Distress and Safety System (GMDSS) is an international satellite system that will soon be the standard and replace the EPIRB system.

■ Marine and weather radio are mandatory for communicating from ship to shore or from ship to ship.

■ Radar, using radio waves, and sonar, using sound waves, are complex navigation aids found on larger sailboats, yachts, and cabin cruisers.

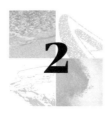

Emergency Packs

An emergency pack should have the vital tools for dealing with misadventure. There are numerous variations on the emergency equipment pack. Some people have one kit with everything; others have separate kits for repair, first-aid, and survival gear. And still others have different kits for different activities. You can buy fully stocked kits from outdoor and marine supply stores, or you can build your own for less money.

I carry one small omni-kit for almost every day trip and sport. It's a survival, first-aid, and repair kit all wrapped into one and stashed in a one-quart freezer bag; you can also use a small stuff sack or zippered bag. It works for day trips whether I'm on the coast surfing or on a two-hour kayak down my local river.

I have separate kits for multiday trips. I have a large first-aid kit, a detailed survival kit, and repair materials that are specific to whatever activity I'm doing. In other words, if I'm going on a surf trip to the Oregon coast with the guys, I might take different things than if I'm taking my family canoe camping in Glacier National Park.

Finally, I have expedition kits for survival, repair, and first aid for long trips, which often stay in my car. These are complex kits in watertight cases designed for extended trips to Baja surfing or two-week river trips with large groups. Some examples of survival and first-aid gear are listed in detail in the rest of this chapter (see pages 17–23).

Don't forget your repair kit; if your boat's broken, you can't get very far! Your gear will largely depend on the type of vessel you're traveling in. A general repair kit includes duct tape, cord, cable ties, wire, and a small pocket tool that contains pliers, wire cutter, screwdrivers, scissors, and a knife. You should have a patch kit, too, but that depends on your craft. Rafts need rubber repair materials. Boats, kayaks, and canoes need plastic, fiberglass, polyester, epoxy, or other type of marine repair sealant, depending on the construction. Sailboats require repair materials for the hull, plus a sewing kit and materials for sail repair.

Survival Gear

Ask experts what to carry for survival kits and you will get several answers. Still, there are some universally accepted survival items you should never be without. For small craft, like kayaks or rafts, you'll need a small kit stowed in a drybag.

■ **Bandages** will treat basic small cuts and scrapes. In general, it's best to have a full first-aid kit as described in the following section.

■ **Extra food and water** above and beyond what you think you will need for the trip—at least an extra quart of water and a few energy bars.

■ **Extra clothing** will depend on the weather. This may be a light rain jacket or a full survival suit, depending on the activity, location, geography, and climate. It's best to have at least one set of dry clothes.

■ **First-aid or duct tape** can be used in a multitude of situations. Waterproof first-aid tape is more durable and easier on the skin, but it costs more than duct tape.

■ A **headlamp,** with extra batteries and bulb, is vital for any activity. It's best to get a waterproof model.

■ A **knife** is important for kayakers, rafters, canoers, and kiteboarders. Get one designed for the sport you're engaged in.

■ **Matches, lighter, or flint** are essential. If you carry matches, use the windproof, waterproof kind and store them in a watertight jar. Flint, also called a metal match, works well to ignite tinder, even when the flint is damp. Fire starter, although not mandatory, helps tremendously when igniting a fire. This can be solid fuel that is shaved into the tinder or fuel tablets.

■ A **chart or map and compass** are universally accepted as the most foolproof means of navigation. You should always have them, even if you carry a GPS (Global Positioning System).

■ **Safety pins** can be used for first-aid and equipment repair in various ways.

■ **Sunscreen,** at least a small tube, should be in your kit.

■ A **PFD** is required for boats in most states and optional for some sports such as sailboarding. Depending on the activity, you may wear it, as in kayaking, or it can be lashed to your boat, such as when you're fishing in a calm lake in good weather.

■ A **multiuse tool** that includes pliers, wire cutters, screwdrivers, scissors, and a knife is essential.

■ A **pump or sponge** is useful for bailing.

■ **Rope or cord** is essential. For swift-water boaters, this is a throw rope. For other sports, you may just bring 25 feet of 5-millimeter accessory cord.

■ A **signal mirror** is important for signaling aircraft or faraway land rescuers.

■ A **water purifier and/or desalinator** can be used to purify fresh water from land or acquire fresh water from seawater, respectively. (Iodine tablets or bleach are alternatives.)

■ A **whistle** is essential for signaling someone on shore, on another boat, or in the water. It will save your voice and is often easier to hear from afar.

Depending on the type and size of your boat as well as the waterway, you may need a larger kit. For example, large oceangoing sailboats will need an extensive survival kit. Without going into detail, here are some additional items you may choose to carry:

- Anchor or sea anchor

- Bailer

- Batteries

- Canned water and food with opener

- Cell phone

- Chemical light sticks

- EPIRB (Emergency Position-Indicating Radio Beacon)

- Fire extinguisher

- Flashlight (underwater)

- Flares or other pyrotechnic signaling devices

- Insect repellent

- Life raft

- Marine radio

- Paddle (extra)

- Pen and paper

- Rescue flag

- Rope (accessory cord, 50 to 100 feet)

- Signal strobe

- Solar still equipment (see the "Potable Water" section)

- Survival suit

- Weather radio

First-Aid Gear

A small first-aid kit is usually all you have room for when kayaking or rafting. Consider keeping it in a resealable freezer bag inside your drybag or tacklebox to make sure the contents stay dry if the container leaks. Usually, small kits contain items to dress wounds and provide some basic medications for common ailments.

- **Anti-inflammatory pain medication** such as ibuprofen helps control pain and limit swelling.

- **Bandages** should be of various sizes.

- **Cloth tape** should be waterproof and plastic coated. It sticks on skin longer than does standard first-aid tape.

- **First-aid ointment** is used on wounds after

cleaning and before the dressing to eliminate bacteria.

■ **First-aid soap** is for washing wounds.

■ **Gauze squares** are used for wound bleeding, cleaning, and dressing. Carry several that are 2 inches and 4 inches square.

■ **Gauze roll,** either 2-inch or 3-inch, is handy for large wounds or for wounds that need a durable dressing, such as one on the leg or arm.

■ **Gloves and pocket mask** are essential to prevent biohazards when performing CPR.

■ **Wound closure strips,** or butterfly bandages, are used to close simple, small, clean cuts.

A larger kit is best for your car or for your boat. Once you've stocked everything on the above list, here are some additional items worth carrying. Remember, you need to know how to use these materials.

■ Ace bandage

■ Antihistamine such as diphenhydramine

■ Large selection of bandages

- Large selection of gauze

- Hydrocortisone cream

- Moleskin

- Needle

- Oral rehydration powder

- Pen, paper, accident report form

- Safety pins

- Splint, wire mesh or metal

- Splinter forceps

- Syringe

- Thermometer

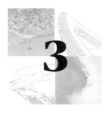

3

Water Survival

Don't Panic!

When disaster strikes, or even when you have a minor mishap, don't panic! Many frightful situations are minor and easily remedied. We hear on the news about major survival incidents at sea or on rivers, but there are many survival success stories that are too easily fixed to make headlines. Above all, don't panic. Keeping your cool is the key to making it through crisis situations.

If you have any warning that disaster may happen, such as rough water or foul weather, take preventive measures immediately. Don your survival suit, warm clothing, and/or foul-weather gear. Put on your PFD. Get your emergency kits ready (survival, first-aid, and repair kits)—especially bailing gear, throw rope, or whatever specific gear the circumstances may call for. Stow all gear, tie down equipment, and secure hatches.

Then, if an accident does occur, take some time to evaluate the current plight, if you can. You might have to do this instantaneously if someone's raft is pinned against a rock, for instance, or your buddy has fallen overboard. Hopefully, you'll have a few minutes to gather your thoughts.

Rescue everyone who's in trouble immediately but cautiously, especially when dealing with a capsized boat or a swamped craft. Once you've rescued them, perform first aid as soon as possible, if needed.

Seek dry land as quickly as possible, or at least head to a sheltered cove. Some hints for rough water:

■ When passing through large swells and waves, approach them at forty degrees.

■ If in a sailboat, put down your daggerboard and reef your sails.

■ Keep your center of gravity low by placing gear or people low and centered in the boat.

■ In a sea kayak, use your rudder.

■ Use extreme caution landing on the shore if you have to pass through breaking surf.

If you have to abandon ship for any reason,

don't forget your survival gear. Gather your emergency kit and life raft. Drink as much fresh water as you can. Activate your EPIRB, send a distress call on the marine radio, and call on your cell or satellite phone if available. Put on your PFD and warmest clothing. Always stay on or near your boat unless it's in danger, such as if it's being crushed by waves, sinking quickly, or on fire.

Once ashore, reassess the situation. Take some time to rest, drink fluids, and regroup.

Then head home immediately and cautiously. If you can hike, paddle, or sail out with your own group, this is usually best. If someone is gravely wounded, you may have to seek help. Waiting for help, even if you can call with a cell phone, will likely take some time, especially in stormy weather and rough seas or if you're in a remote location. This is why you should always have reserves of food and water, a dry change of clothes, an emergency kit with survival gear, and extra energy reserves.

Overboard

Sooner or later, you'll get dunked. Hopefully this won't be a major deal and you can swim back to your boat. But in some circumstances you may have only minutes to initiate lifesaving survival measures, depending on how tired you are, how cold the water is, and how bad the weather and water conditions are. Follow some basic steps:

■ Signal by waving, shouting, shining a light, and/or using a whistle. You must notify your partners on the boat immediately that you've gone into the drink. They may be continuing on their way and get out of earshot or whistle distance in a matter of seconds.

■ Conserve energy by using one of several survival swim/float techniques discussed in the next couple of pages.

■ Use clothing to help you float. Tie knots in your pant legs, inflate them by pulling them out of the water, then squeeze the waist shut and tie it with a belt to hold in air. You can also blow air into your shirt. It will get trapped in the shoulders and provide some flotation.

■ If your boat is swamped in swift water, keep the canoe, kayak, or raft in front and downstream of you. Hold the stern with the bow downstream until you get to calm water or an eddy. (See the illustration on page 40.)

■ For offshore vessels, you should have an

inflatable life raft, survival provisions, an EPIRB, and a survival suit.

Make a decision whether to swim to shore, swim to your boat, or wait for help. This depends mostly on weather and water conditions, the distance you are from dry land, and the likelihood that someone (a partner or rescue professional) can rescue you. If your boat is nearby, this is one of the best piece of survival gear you can have. Even if it has capsized, you can sit on top and get out of the water. You will also need it—and all the gear that's stowed in or lashed on it—for the trip back to safety.

Some specific swim survival techniques include the survival float, heat-escape-lessening position, huddle, and swift-water float.

Survival Float

The survival float allows you to use as little energy as possible. Take a breath, then float facedown with your arms extended. Relax and use your feet sparingly to stay upright. When you need a breath, slowly lift your head from the water, take a breath while treading with your arms and legs, then relax into the water again. Practice this in a swimming pool. The most difficult part is learning to mentally relax enough to float facedown in water.

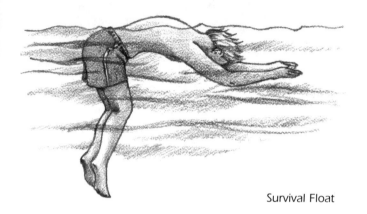

Survival Float

Heat-Escape-Lessening Position (HELP)

The HELP position allows you to save energy and retain heat while wearing a PFD. From a sitting position, keep your head out of the water. Cross your hands in front of your chest. Bring your knees up to your chest.

Huddle

If you're with one or more persons, the huddle position keeps you all together and minimizes heat loss. Face together in a circle, and stay as close as possible to your partner(s) for warmth. With several people, put a child, the coldest person, or the one who can't swim in the middle.

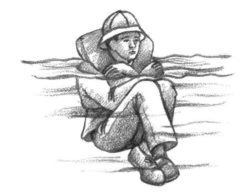

HELP

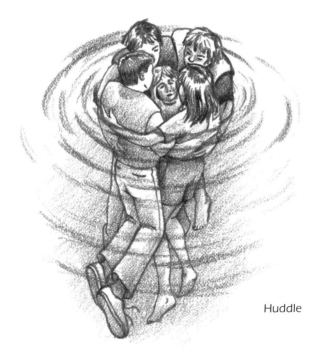

Huddle

Swift-Water Swim

The swift-water swim position allows you to fend off rocks and logs as you make your way through rapids to calm water. In a sitting position, face downstream. Keep your legs out in front of you and near the surface to fend off rocks and logs; use your arms to swim and maneuver.

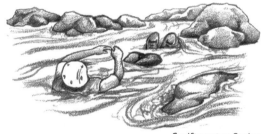

Swift-water Swim

Signaling

If you're in dire need of help, signal, signal, signal. Attracting the attention of rescuers immediately could mean the difference between life and death. If your potential rescuers are nearby, you can signal for help immediately by shouting, waving your arms, blowing a whistle, or shining a light. Remember, they may quickly travel out of shouting or whistling distance. If

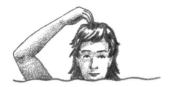

All Clear

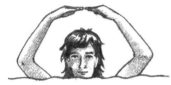

All Clear (OK)

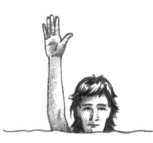

Assistance
Needed

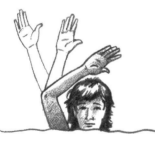

Resuscitation
Case or Oxygen
Needed

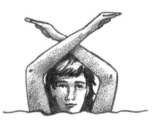

Submerged
Swimmer

Lifeguard Hand Signals

you're at a beach, you can use lifeguard hand
signals to alert rescuers on the shore.

■ Two hands clasped overhead, or one hand
  touching your head, means "Everything's
  okay."

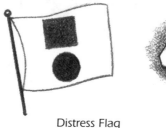

Distress Flag

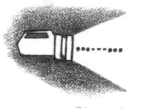

Distress Strobe

■ One hand straight up or waving means "Need help."

■ Two hands crossed overhead means "Swimmer submerged."

If on a boat, you should have other devices available. Activate flares or other pyrotechnic signaling devices. Put out a distress flag (orange with a black circle and square) during the day, or rescue lights (that automatically flash SOS) at night. You can also fly your boat's flag upside down, another universal sign of distress. Use sea dye, smoke signals, or chemical light sticks. International code flags N (November) and C (Charlie) also signal distress. For more distant rescuers—and especially to signal aircraft—use a signal mirror.

If you're distant from rescuers or are in a

remote location, you'll probably be relying on portable electronics such as a cell or satellite phone, marine radio, or EPIRB. With a phone, dial 911. If you have a marine radio, channel 16 (2182 kHz SSB) is the emergency channel monitored by the U.S. Coast Guard. If you have an EPIRB, remember to turn it on.

Emergency Navigation

Navigation is a complex skill that takes formal instruction then lots of experience to master. I won't even try to do more than provide an introduction. The basis for navigation is a nautical chart or a land map and a compass. A chart for waterways has depths marked and connected by lines; it also shows ports, buoys, land markers, and other information needed for compass navigation. A map for land navigation has topographic lines that show elevation of the land, geographic features like waterfalls, and human-made features such as dams, as well as other information. You can get charts and maps for nearly every navigable waterway or land area in the world.

To accompany a chart in navigable waterways, use a pilot—a reference book to waterways—and a nautical almanac describing historical

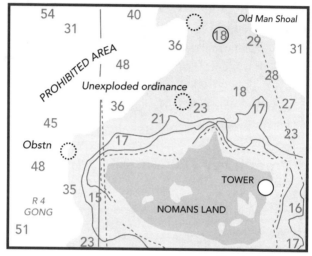

Nautical Chart

weather and water patterns. These list detailed directions to various routes, including potential hazards, both permanent and seasonal, as well as typical weather and water patterns. You should also make use of channel markers, lateral aids, and regulatory markers.

Compasses come in a variety of forms: electronic, manual, wristwatch. Learn how to use one before you set out, and practice in water you know well.

GPS is especially useful. These units also take lots of experience to master. They might be handheld units or larger bridge-mounted models. You need a chart or map with GPS coordinates, or way points, to navigate with a GPS.

Dead reckoning, a rather old technique for navigation, is recommended for emergencies only.

Remember, always abide by navigational rules and maritime law.

Without reviewing all the elements of compass or GPS navigation, here are some helpful definitions and hints:

■ **Magnetic north** is the direction a compass points to.

■ **True north** is the direction of the North Pole, and the direction of north on a map or chart.

■ **Declination** is the deviation between magnetic and true north.

■ **Field bearing** is a compass reading based on magnetic north.

■ **Map bearing** is a map or chart reading based on true north.

■ Keep the manual for your compass or GPS with you so that you can use it correctly. Keep it in a watertight freezer bag or watertight case with your map, chart, or GPS.

- An altimeter can be useful on inland water-ways.

- Practice your navigation skills in known waters. Keep track of your position as you sail.

- Carry extra batteries for your GPS and store it in a watertight case.

Boat Problems

There are many accidents that can occur to your boat. It's been said, in fact, that you're not on an adventure until something breaks! Generally, the more complicated and high tech, the more likely it is that the boat, or something on it, can break. Try to be prepared for mishaps. Here are some common ones.

Boat Repair

You should be well versed and practiced in boat repair. It's not something you should be doing for the first time when afloat. You must have the correct materials and tools. For a kayak, canoe, or boat, you will need epoxy, polyester, fiberglass, plastic, or a similar marine repair material. For a raft, a rubber patch kit and pump are essential. Sailors should bring a sewing kit and patch materials for sails.

Capsized

If you capsize, you might have to be Hercules to get some boats right-side up. For rafts or sailboats that are not self-righting, stand atop the upturned craft, tie a rope on one side, then, using your body as counterweight, flip the boat. Make sure you don't bonk your head on a rock or log when the boat flips.

Swamped

If a canoe or kayak is swamped, you can sometimes use a bailer to evacuate the water or

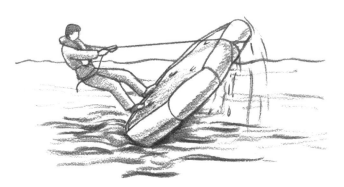

Righting Raft

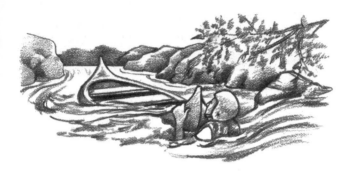

Holding Swamped Canoe

another person's boat to roll the canoe or kayak and pour it out. If you need to guide a swamped canoe or kayak to shore or if you're in rapids, get behind the boat and hold the stern. The boat will lead you downstream until you can safely guide it ashore.

Towing

If you need to tow another boat, use caution in rough weather or water. Use a towline, keep a good distance between boats, and go slow. The distance between canoes, kayaks, or small boats should be around 25 feet. Make sure the line is fastened on a cleat but easy to remove; if not, have a knife handy to cut the line.

Fire

Always be cautious of fire on larger boats, especially those that have galleys. Fires occur most often when cooking. Use precautions to avoid fire and carry a fire extinguisher.

Potable Water

Most people know that you won't last longer than a few days without drinking water. Your emergency kit should have at least a quart of water; better is a day's supply (two to four quarts per person, depending on conditions). Not everyone is able to have so much in reserve, however, and it often isn't practical in small kayaks and such.

At Sea

When at sea, you should carry a portable desalinator. These handheld pumps remove salt from seawater and yield fresh drinking water. This takes some time; if the water is thick with debris or seaweed, you may need to strain it first through a paper towel or bandanna.

Hint: Never drink salt water. Instead of being absorbed, the salt water draws fresh water out of your body and causes severe dehydration in a matter of minutes.

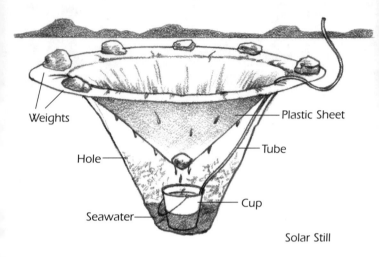

Weights — Plastic Sheet

Hole — Tube

Seawater — Cup

Solar Still

If you don't have a desalinator, you should have materials to construct a solar still for an emergency: a thin sheet of clear plastic, a small cup, and a flexible tube. Place salt water in the bottom of a life raft. In the middle, place the empty cup and put one end of your tube in it. Then spread your clear plastic sheet over the raft and place a weight in the middle of the sheet directly over the cup. Line the sheet with rocks, logs, or other objects to weight it. Place the other end of the tube outside the sheet so you can drink from the cup without removing the sheet. As the sun heats up the seawater, only water evaporates, leaving the salt behind.

When the water condenses on the sheet then collects into the cup, it has no salt in it. This is an extremely slow method for distilling fresh water—it sometimes yields only a cup a day. Use this only as an emergency backup method for procuring fresh water when you are stranded at sea with no other recourse.

In Fresh Water

If you're on inland lakes or rivers, you'll have a supply of freshwater. It should be purified, however, since many freshwater sources are contaminated with bacteria, protozoans, and viruses. Although there are several methods for purifying water, only two are realistic for most adventurers.

The quickest and easiest in a survival situation is to use either iodine tablets or household bleach. One or two tablets of iodine will purify a quart bottle of water. Iodine tastes bad, so you can buy a second tablet that neutralizes the taste. With chlorine bleach, use five to ten drops to purify a quart of water. The advantage of iodine is that the tablets are easy to carry; chlorine bleach needs to be in a watertight durable plastic jar. Keep in mind that a few encapsulated protozoan spores are partially or completely resistant to some chemical treatment.

Alternatively, many freshwater enthusiasts carry a mechanical purifier. A hand-pump purifier comes in several sizes, is simple to use, and achieves total purification. These usually have three components: a filter for large pathogens, iodine to kill viruses that are too small to be filtered, and charcoal to remove the chemical taste. Be cautious when you buy a hand pump. Some units are filters only that don't totally purify because they lack the chemical on the filter. If the water is hazy, filled with debris, or brackish, you may need to strain it with a bandanna or T-shirt first before purifying it mechanically or with chemicals.

Boiling seawater to remove salt or boiling fresh water to kill pathogens is too laborious and requires too much extra equipment—such as a stove, fuel, and cooking pot—to be useful in a survival situation unless you have no other alternative and you're able to carry a cook set with your survival gear.

Fishing

Obtaining food when in a survival situation is relatively low priority if you expect rescue within a day. It can be dangerous, even fatal, to eat poisonous fish. Hopefully you have some survival rations or at least an energy bar. Most people do okay without food for a day.

If you're at sea or in a wilderness riverine environment and have the appropriate fishing tackle, you can fish. If you've had advanced survival training, you can construct a fishing pole from a tree limb, fishhook, and twine. There are also several methods for creating fish traps from limbs and rocks. When at sea, make sure you carry and know how to use fish identification cards: Several kinds of fish are poisonous.

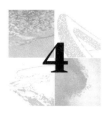

First Aid

One More Time: Don't Panic

Okay, sometimes first-aid situations happen. Remember, don't panic. The sight of blood can be scary, but with a little soap and water you might find it's only a tiny cut. Before initiating first aid, you should be trained in a water- or outdoor-oriented course that provides instruction on basic wound care and splinting sprains and fractures. Also, a cardiopulmonary resuscitation (CPR) course is vital. Generally, you shouldn't attempt CPR unless you know what you're doing. Most courses, including those by the American Heart Association and those endorsed by the Wilderness Medical Society, teach the primary survey and the secondary survey.

Primary Survey

The primary survey basically takes you through the ABCDE exam. Airway: Check and clear.

Breathing: Look, listen, and feel. Circulation: Check for signs of heartbeat such as breathing, coughing, chest movement, or a pulse (if trained). Disability: Check for a major injury disabling the victim. Exposure: Remember to prevent hypothermia and other environmental illnesses while you are assessing, treating, and evacuating the person.

Secondary Survey

The secondary survey is a detailed total-body inspection of the injured person to make sure you don't miss wounds.

Major Injury

As with most first aid, you need formal training to treat major shock and trauma. *Trauma* is a term used for any injury, but usually refers to large, significant wounds. *Shock* is a general term for distress. It may be due to cardiopulmonary arrest, head or spine injury, major bleeding, heatstroke, hypothermia, near drowning, or a host of other medical problems. Remember: For major head or spine injuries, don't move the victim. He or she needs total immobilization on a back board with a cervical collar to prevent worsening of the condition.

CPR Refresher

If someone isn't breathing or shows no signs of circulation, you may need to start CPR. The American Heart Association has a stepwise plan for you to follow. All I can do is offer a very quick reminder; you will need to have had formal training on these techniques. It's very difficult to do CPR in the water. If you can lay the victim on a surfboard or in a dinghy, for example, you may be able to float alongside or straddle the person, respectively.

■ Shout and make contact with the person to see if he or she is alert.

■ Yell for assistance from your buddies.

■ Gently place the person on his or her back— unless there's any chance of a head or spine injury, in which case don't move the victim.

■ Don't forget to wear gloves. You should have them in your first-aid supplies.

■ Clean the mouth with your finger and straighten the neck and airway with the chin lift. Use the jaw thrust technique (without moving the patient's neck) if you're worried about a spinal injury.

■ If the patient isn't breathing, start with two rescue breaths using your CPR mask. Use a bag-mask ventilator if you have one and are trained in its use. There are some circumstances in which respiratory support is vital, including near drowning and submersion.

■ Look for signs of the heart beating: normal breathing, coughing, chest movement, and warm skin. Check for a pulse, if you're trained.

■ If you determine that the heart isn't beating, start chest compressions at one hundred per minute, pausing for two breaths after fifteen compressions. The compression point is at the center of the chest, right between the nipples.

■ Attach an automated external defibrillator (AED), if you're trained in its use and have one available. These are becoming more common on cruise ships, lifeguard stations, Coast Guard ships, and at many public places.

Wounds

You'll get cut, sooner or later. Wounds are common and, fortunately, usually easy to care for. Blood doesn't clot well in water, so with a major wound, get out of the water as soon as possible.

Clean cuts and scrapes with clean water, preferably not seawater or unpurified river water. Wash with first-aid or camp soap. Apply pressure for several minutes to stop the bleeding. When the wound is clean and the bleeding is stanched, spread a thin layer of first-aid ointment over the wound to prevent infection. Cover with a bandage, gauze, and/or waterproof first-aid tape. For small cuts, you may be able to use butterfly bandages.

Fishhooks

If you fish, it's only a matter of time before you get jabbed with a hook. There is no painless way to remove one in the field. It's best to let your local emergency room remove it. If you're in the boonies, however, you can try to remove it yourself (or with a partner's help).

If the barb is totally buried in your skin, you have two options. First, you can try to back out the hook. Tie a string or ribbon around the hook at the bend. Then gently pull on the string while holding the hook eye against your skin.

Alternatively, advance the hook through

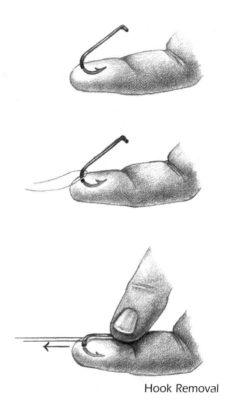

Hook Removal

your skin on the other side of your finger. Then, with pliers, snip off the tip of the hook (including the barb) and back out the remainder of the hook the way it came in.

After removal, wash the skin thoroughly and have your doctor check it.

Extremity Injury

Next to cuts and scrapes, twisted ankles or shoulder sprains are probably the most common injury for watersports enthusiasts. Watersports use upper and lower extremities for maneuvers, so ankles, knees, hips, shoulders, elbows, and wrists are frequently injured. The most difficult assessment in the field can be distinguishing a simple injury from a broken bone. Any time you see a deformity, hear a crunch or pop, have an open wound, or are unable to use the affected arm or leg, you should suspect a broken bone or dislocation.

Treatment uses the RICE method: rest, ice, compression, elevation. Anti-inflammatory pills will help with pain and swelling.

For significant injuries, you'll need to make a splint. Pad the affected leg or arm using clothing. Then, using a splint from your first-aid kit, or an improvised one from sticks or paddles, immobilize the arm or leg. Avoid tying the splint so tight that fingers or toes go numb or get cold. For an arm injury, after you make a splint, use a sling to support the arm from the neck, then tie it to the chest with a swath. For a leg injury, after you splint the leg, you can use boat paddles for crutches.

Hypothermia

Hypothermia usually occurs if you fall into frigid water. Initially you feel cold and shiver—that's a normal response. When you lose core body heat—which can happen very quickly in cold water—you become dizzy and tired and can have impaired judgment and coordination; you may have trouble swimming or following directions. Eventually you display confusion and slurred speech and stop shivering; at this point, you're unable to swim to safety. The best treatment and prevention: Get out of the water as soon as possible (or rescue the victim) and change into warm dry clothing! Eating food and drinking fluids will help, too.

Dehydration

Dehydration often occurs without a person knowing it. With some adventure sports, it can be difficult to carry and drink fresh water—and sometimes we forget to drink fluids regularly. In addition, the body loses water through sweating, even in the water. Dehydration usually starts with headache, dizziness, and thirst.

When dehydration occurs, replace fluids with water, a sports drink, or oral rehydration solution. Never drink seawater or urine; this will further dehydrate you.

Sunburn

We've all had a bad sunburn at one time or another. It's unfortunately more common in water activities than with most other sports. The problem is that if we're feeling cool water on our skin, we don't feel the heat radiation of the sun—and sunscreen washes off quickly. There's also a delay between the time we're exposed to the sun and when the pain of a burn starts; it sneaks up on us. Snorkelers, skin divers, and surfers are particularly vulnerable since they tend to be uncovered and directly exposed, but they don't notice the hot sun because of the cool water on their skin.

The best option is to cover all exposed skin with a wetsuit, rash guard, or sun protective clothing (as discussed in chapter 1 in "Personal Protective Clothing") and to wear waterproof sunblock that's equal to or greater than 25 SPF. Surfproof sunblock may stay on skin longer. Basically, the waxier the lotion, the longer it adheres to skin. If you get sunburned, aloe vera lotion will help with pain and redness.

Aquatic Animals

Aquatic animals are beautiful—but at the same time potentially lethal. They won't harm us so long as we give them a wide berth. Nontoxic animal bites and stings are treated with good wound care as described in that section. For toxic animals, use the guidelines below.

Jellyfish, coral, and anemones can sting, causing a rash, skin irritation, and even some systemic symptoms, including nausea, vomiting, dizziness, chills, and bodyaches. Rinse with seawater, not fresh water, then pour vinegar on the skin to neutralize the toxin. Baking soda, rubbing alcohol, or meat tenderizer may work, too. After the stinging subsides, the small cysts can be removed by applying shaving cream and shaving with a razor.

For puncture by a sea urchin, starfish, or stingray spine, place the injured area in hot water (nonscalding) to neutralize the toxin. Carefully remove the spine, then clean the wound as described in "Wounds" on pages 50–51.

Near Drowning

Drowning is something everyone respects, and with good reason. It's the most common cause of accidental death in watersports. It's often accompanied by head trauma or prolonged submersion. Learn to swim, use a helmet, and wear your PFD!

If you're at the scene of a near drowning, try to reach the person or toss a PFD or throw rope. Tow the person to a boat or shore immediately. The chief focus is on respiratory resuscitation. Many near-drowning victims survive if CPR is started right away. Remember to remove wet clothes and replace them with warm, dry garments. Be cautious of vomiting.

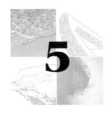

5

Special Circumstances

Land Survival

All water enthusiasts should know that survival on water is sometimes only half the battle. Once you get ashore, you may need to employ land survival techniques until help arrives or while you hike out to your car. Although not the focus of this book, there are books listed in appendix A that cover these techniques, including land navigation with a map and compass, procuring water from the sea or purifying fresh water, and other survival issues. Two items—building a fire and finding shelter—are critical to land survival, however, and are worth mentioning.

A fire can be used to keep you warm, cook food, dry out wet clothes, boil water, distill seawater, make a smoke signal, and provide light. A small campfire can help lift spirits, too. Keep your fire small. Start it in a small fire pit, dry streambed, or on rocks. You'll need some type of fire starter such as dry matches, a lighter, or flint and knife blade, also called a metal match. Start with dry tinder, small sticks, needles, or dry leaves. Add layers of larger sticks and logs slowly. Remember to squelch coals with water and spread the cold, wet ashes when you leave your fire.

Numerous methods for building a shelter will keep you dry and warm when on land. It largely depends on where you are and what materials you may have brought ashore with you.

The quickest shelter is to use your capsized boat, whether it's a sailboat, canoe, kayak, or raft. If you capsize at sea or in a large lake or stream, you should never leave your craft; it's your best piece of survival equipment. You can sit atop an upturned sailboat or raft and stay out of the cold water. The trick is getting it ashore if you have no motor or paddles. Use caution dragging an upturned boat through surf, rocks, or swift water. Once ashore, you'll have your boat for shelter as well as most of your gear, hopefully. Even a surfboard can keep the rain off when used as part of a basic shelter. With a few sticks or some rope, you can prop your boat up on one end and crawl underneath to get out of the rain or cold.

If your boat isn't available, use whatever materials you have with you or can find on land. Flotsam (debris floating in the water, like driftwood) or jetsam (equipment and materials that came from your capsized boat) can be used for shelter with some improvisation. The quickest and easiest shelter is to string a tarp across some logs or rocks. If you're in a forest, you can improvise a lean-to using downed sticks, tree limbs and boughs, and sometimes tree wells. On the seashore, driftwood can be stacked to form a shelter. If you're in an area with large rocks, stack them to make walls and cover the top with a tarp or sticks.

Open-Ocean Survival

Open-ocean survival is a gigantic subject that spans entire lifetimes of some survival experts. It can only be briefly highlighted here. Survival depends on your skill and specialty equipment—be well prepared! You can find gear at marine or boat supply stores.

For open-ocean vessels, you need a full tool kit, repair materials, and the skill to fix damaged sails, hulls, or engines. You need bailing equipment and a bilge pump. Fire prevention at sea is paramount in any vessel with a motor, kitchen, or heater. A fully stocked expedition first-aid kit and extensive knowledge of first-aid in remote areas is crucial for treating illnesses and injuries.

You must have a life raft and survival suit to prevent hypothermia. Emergency rations of food and water, especially canned or bottled water, are a must for prolonged survival. Fishing tackle is important for procuring food in extended situations. Signal devices, as outlined under "Signaling," are crucial, especially an EPIRB, satellite phone, or marine radio. You should be highly skilled at open-ocean navigation and have the necessary tools for it.

Dive Medicine

Scuba diving is a worldwide sport that explores the fascinating but dangerous underwater world. Diving health problems are also beyond the scope of this book, but it's worth mentioning several common conditions.

Dysbarism is a general term for illnesses caused by a change in pressure. For example, when you dive underwater, the higher pressure can cause ear, sinus, tooth, and lung problems. Pulmonary overpressurization syndrome is a condition in which expanding air injures the small air sacs of the lungs. With an arterial gas embolism, air bubbles in the bloodstream get trapped in the small capillary beds of the heart.

Decompression sickness, called the bends, occurs when you surface and bubbles of air form in your bloodstream and tissues. Symptoms include joint pain, muscle aches, and dizziness, among others.

For health-related issues regarding diving, check with a detailed text. To get a diving card, you'll also need to get a physical exam by your doctor. Check with the Divers Alert Network hot line at (919) 684–8111 or boot up www.diversalertnetwork.org.

Safety Tips for Surf Riders

Action sports can be an adrenaline rush, whether it's riding waves or running rapids. Surfers, kiteboarders, windsurfers, and surf or whitewater kayakers have one chief thing in common: They generally carry little to no rescue gear, mostly because there's little extra room on their person or in their boat or board. Often they carry only the bare essentials: wetsuit, helmet, cord, knife, and PFD.

If you carry one item, it should be 30 feet of heavy cord. This is especially important for

Windsurfers and kiters so that you can repair lines or tow another person who can't make it to shore. If you're kayaking or kiteboarding, carry a knife to cut lines if they become tangled or caught on flotsam and you're unable to get them unstuck; it should be sheathed and designed for the respective sport. Above all, never abandon your board or boat. This is your primary means of flotation other than a PFD.

Wetsuits are the key to protection against hypothermia. The suit should be warm enough for the conditions if you break down and need to spend lots of time in the water repairing gear, swimming, or helping another person. A good rule: Always dress a bit warmer than conditions call for. For wetsuits, the thickness and length of the sleeves and legs vary widely; see "Personal Protective Clothing" in chapter 1 for more information. Depending on the conditions, consider neoprene gloves, booties, and hat.

Helmets designed for watersports are important, as mentioned in "Personal Protective Clothing." Goggles protect from sunlight as well as water splashing. Most goggles designed specifically for watersports float, provide good peripheral vision, and are comfortable and secure. Polarized lenses decrease reflected glare

and therefore lessen the definition and sub-
tleties of the water. Water spots on the lenses
can decrease visibility, too; some surf riders use
lens coatings to help prevent this. To keep
water out of the nose, some windsurfers and
kayakers have had good luck using nose clips
like those designed for swimming. Foam
earplugs provide some protection for ears.
Remember though that all this headgear will
blunt your senses. Valuable senses such as
peripheral vision, smell, and hearing can be significantly decreased.

Using a PFD for surfing is rare, and for windsurfing and kiteboarding it's controversial.
Windsurfers and kiters are exempt in most
states from the law requiring boaters to carry
PFDs. Wearing a PFD makes it more difficult to
Windsurf but provides flotation if you have a
problem. They are perhaps most useful to those
who are learning.

For surfing, kiteboarding, and especially
windsurfing—a highly technical, gear-laden
sport—all parts should be checked regularly. If
you're surfing, the board and its fins should be
strong and sealed, and the leash should be in
good condition. In windsurfing, the sail, boom,
universal joint, and ropes should be in excellent

condition and replaced readily if wearing. For kiting, check your leashes and lines for wear and tear.

Swift-Water Rescue

Swift-water rescue—a situation encountered by kayakers, rafters, canoers, and boaters running rapids—is another specialty area requiring skills and techniques beyond the scope of this book. Swimming through holes, waves, ledges, rapids, falls, and strainers (logjams and debris) is technical; you need skill at negotiating rapids, swift water, and even waterfalls. You need a durable watercraft as well as lots of flotation and specialty equipment.

Specialty safety equipment for whitewater or surf kayaks includes a spray skirt. Canoes usually have air bladders for flotation. Rafts need oar-locks, a frame kit, and a patch kit for rubber. Gear includes PFDs, helmets, wetsuits, paddles, and a hand bailing pump designed for swift-water use.

The chief means of rescuing a stranded swift-water boater is the throw rope. This is a water-proof line coiled or stuffed into a bag. From shore or from another boat, the rescuer throws the line to the stranded boater. A knife is usually carried when working with rope. If a rope becomes taut or entangles a person, cutting it is sometimes the only recourse. To throw a throw bag, timing and practice are just as important as strength and distance. Hold the bag with the open end down. Take out the first few feet and hold it. Then throw the bag with an even, steady toss. Aim just upstream from your target.

It's worth your time to learn more complex rescue techniques such as belays, anchors, double lines, or complicated extractions with pulleys or prusiks. These are used when righting a boat, retrieving a boat that's pinned against a rock, or retrieving a runaway craft.

Appendix A

For Further Reading

There are full books that cover nearly every section in this little book. If you find you're deficient in a particular area, supplement your knowledge with a full-length text. Below are perhaps the most useful books.

American Red Cross. *Lifeguarding Today*. St. Louis, MO: Mosby Lifeline, 1995.

Backer, Howard, et al. *Wilderness First Aid: Emergency Care for Remote Locations.* Sudbury, MA: Jones and Bartlett, 1998.

Beilan, Michael. *Your Offshore Doctor: A Manual of Medical Self-Sufficiency at Sea,* 2nd ed. Dobbs Ferry, NY: Sheridan House, 1996.

Brewster, B. C. (ed.) *The United States Lifesaving Association Manual of Open Water Lifesaving.* Englewood Cliffs, NJ: Brady/Prentice Hall, 1995.

Craighead, Frank Jr., and John J. *How to Survive on Land and Sea,* 4th ed. Washington, D.C.: Naval Institute Press, 1984.

Forgey, William. *Wilderness Medicine: Beyond First Aid,* 5th ed. Guilford, CT: Globe Pequot, 1999.

Walbridge, Charles, and Wayne Sundmacher. *Whitewater Rescue Manual: New Techniques for Canoeists, Kayakers, and Rafters.* Camden, ME: Ragged Mountain, 1995.

Weiss, Eric A. *A Comprehensive Guide to Wilderness and Travel Medicine,* 2nd ed. Oakland, CA: Adventure Medical Kits, 1997.

Wilkerson, James A., M.D. (ed.) *Medicine for Mountaineering and Other Wilderness Activities,* 4th ed. Seattle: The Mountaineers, 1992.

Wiseman, John. *The SAS Survival Handbook.* London: HarperCollins, 1999.

Appendix B

Float Plan

1. Person Reporting Overdue

Name _____

Address _____

Phone _____

2. Description of Boat

Registration Number _____

Length _____

Make _____

Type _____

Hull Color _____

Trim Color _____

Fuel Capacity _____

Engine Type _____

Number of Engines _____

Distinguishing Features _____

3. Operator of Boat

Name _____

Age _____

Health _____

Phone _____

Address _____

Operator's Experience _____

4. Survival Equipment

PFDs (number) _____

Smoke Signals _____

Paddles _____

Raft _____

Flares _____

Flashlight _____

Water _____

EPIRB _____

Mirror _____

Food _____

Anchor _____

5. Marine Radio

Type _____

Frequencies _____

6. Trip Expectations

Departure Location _____

Date _____

Time _____

Arrival Location _____

Date _____

Time _____

Call Coast Guard or local authority if not
arrived by:

Date _____

Time _____

Phone _____

7. Vehicle Description

License Number _____

Make _____

Model _____

Color _____

Where Parked? _____

8. Persons on Board

Name _____

Age _____

Phone _____

Medical Conditions _____

Name _____

Age _____

Phone _____

Medical Conditions _____

Name _____

Age _____

Phone _____

Medical Conditions _____

9. Remarks_____

_____

_____

_____

_____

_____

Index

About the Author

Christopher Van Tilburg is a physician and the author of six outdoor books, including *Backcountry Snowboarding, Backcountry Ski Oregon,* and *Canyoneering: Beginning to Advanced Techniques.* For several years, he wrote a column called "Ask Dr. Chris" in the international windsurfing magazine *Wind Tracks.* He's currently a board member of the Wilderness Medical Society, the adventure sports editor of *Wilderness Medicine Letter,* and a member of Mountain Rescue Association. He works as an emergency physician in Hood River, Oregon, and as a mountain doctor on Mount Hood, Oregon. He has windsurfed, surfed, kayaked, canoed, and kiteboarded around the world. His home break is the Columbia River Gorge in Oregon, where he teaches his daughters, Skylar and Avrie, to swim.